A Golden Nugget Way Of Life

Rita A. Ramsey

To order additional copies of this book, contact:
Xlibris Corporation
1-888-795-4274
www.Xlibris.com
Orders@Xlibris.com
86242

Author's Contact Information

ritaaramsey@aol.com
635 Sidney Drive
Lake Helen, FL 32744

INTRODUCTION

No one can go according to "Don't eat this or don't eat that because you will never live up to it!

My book will never try to give you guilt trips, but it will take a stand against indulging eating in excess.

"Fill my cup Lord, I lift it up Lord, come and quench this thirsting of my soul, bread of heaven, feed me 'til I want no more, fill my cup, fill it up and make me whole."

I am not going to fill these pages with recipes, as there are many magazines with recipes of every kind. However, I do have many of my own, and I will be happy to supply you with my favorite recipes and shakes, as well as my mom's favorites, with a new twist, less fat and still tasty! FREE! Wow, do I ever have a good one for banana bread! I do love to make homemade bread.—Well, I got that gift from my mother and it is my favorite thing to do.

I lost 30 pounds, August 01, 2005 to August 01, 2006 by changing my eating habits. You can do it too! Stop thinking that you are going to lose 30 lbs over night; it won't happen and if it did, it would slowly creep right back and you would encounter the Yo-Yo syndrome—up and down! My goal—was one year of consistently changing the way I thought, *correcting what I bought from the grocery store. A good thing to remember is, if you don't purchase it, you won't be tempted to eat it, 'cause it's still on the shelf at the store.*

My book has been laying on the shelf collecting dust and suddenly I realized that perhaps I can help others by getting it published. Proof is in the pudding, as my mother used to say, and it is now 2010, five years later and I have maintained this way of life and kept the 30 lbs. off!

I dedicate this book to all my children, grandchildren and great grandchildren! Charles, Brian, Steve, Tom, Teri, Thad, Barbara, Bonnie, Greg . . . Thane, Trent, Ivan, Dane, Joel, Adam, Ali, Rachel and Livvie; Rhett and Brian, Cody and Taylor, Ian, Andrew and Tristan . . . Seth, Aaron and Summer, Dominique and Kearsten, Jakoa and Silas.

"Realize, faith without works is dead" <u>*James 2:20.*</u>

Many times a day our hunger clock causes us to rush to the cupboard and refrigerator and without counting the costs, we grab that macadamia nut cookie or leftover fried chicken and consume it with a bottle of soda pop or perhaps, in some people's lives, a can of beer. My, my, we fail to realize all the calories we are emptying into this barrel called our stomach, which is only as large as our fist! I know you probably know what Dunlap Disease is—and if you don't, it means your stomach has dun lapped over from putting too much in it!

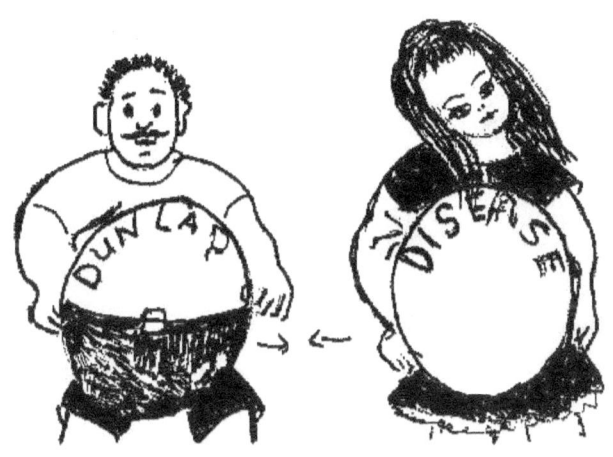

Since visiting Mom's kitchen growing up, we now hang onto habits that reared their ugly head from childhood. Actually, it seemed okay while we were little, because we ran and played hard and oops, all the calories were demolished, but now we spend hours watching TV and our lives have become more complacent in many ways. Let's face it—today's lifestyles are not the same and all this fast paced living has amounted to grabbing a hamburger at McDonalds or some fast food restaurant.

Today, I want you to just lean back on your chair and take a look at *"What is making you Fat."* Let's get back to the basics!!

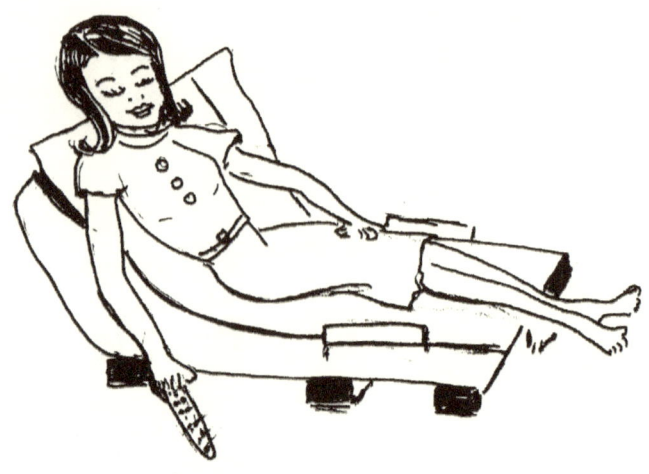

To help you and your family realize *"What's Unhealthy"* for you, let's just take a look inside your refrigerator. You know what the problem is, and that it can be solved! Yes! I want you to spend some time with me today inside your fridge as well as mine.

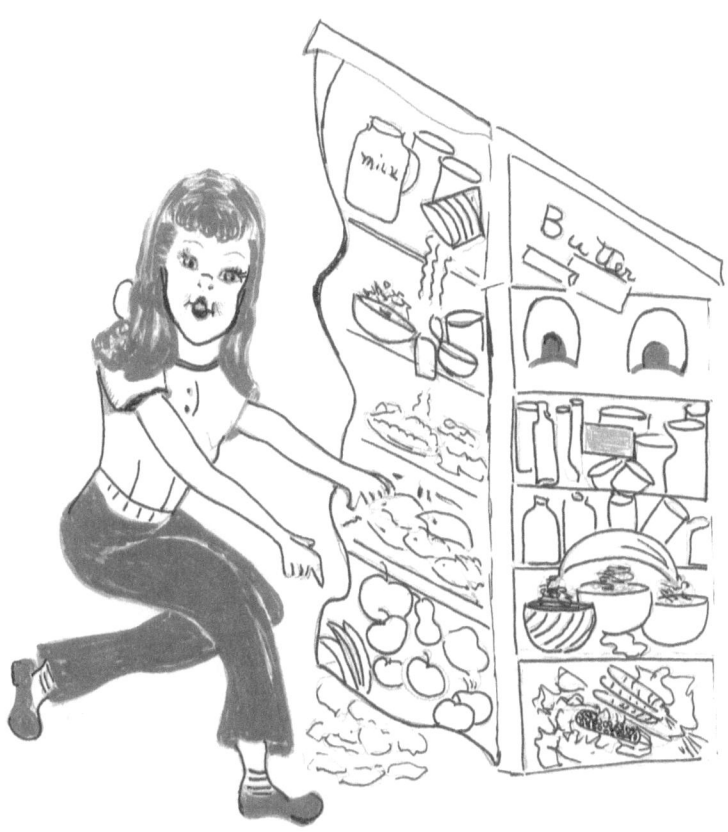

Top shelf—hmmm, milk, a gallon of whole milk. Fat analysis will shock you—I'll let you read the label. 5 grams of fat! Realize if you purchase 1% you have reduced your fat intake. That's a good start! No, I'm not going to buy any more whole milk. A good rule to remember is to never eat or drink anything that is over 2.5 fat content. Oh, here's a tub of sour cream. Now I really do not like the taste of sour cream if it is fat free, but an alternative measure would be to get the reduced fat sour cream, which actually tastes just as good and it is not going to put a rubber tire around your waist.

At the present moment, I am just dealing with fat content. Now, I see some whipped butter. Such a pretty container and such deceit inside . . . Salted, sweet cream. Total saturated fat is 5 grams. Three grams higher than our new rule; Nothing higher than 2.5. An alternative would be "I can't believe it's not butter" or any of the margarines which mainly list 2.0 grams of fat. By the way, the butter contains saturated fat ; that means it's hard fat and very bad for our arteries and heart. Be sure, though, when you buy butter or margarine, that it does not contain trans fats.

Yes, God knew what He was doing when He gave us the dairy cow and the only thing He did not add was chocolate syrup to the milk, but haven't we decided to place a tablespoon of saturated butter on our toast ('cause it tastes so good) and gobble it down with a glass or two of whole milk? The bottom line is, if you can't give up butter and whole milk, then become that temperate person and reduce the amounts you use to 1/2 teaspoon on bread and a six ounce glass of

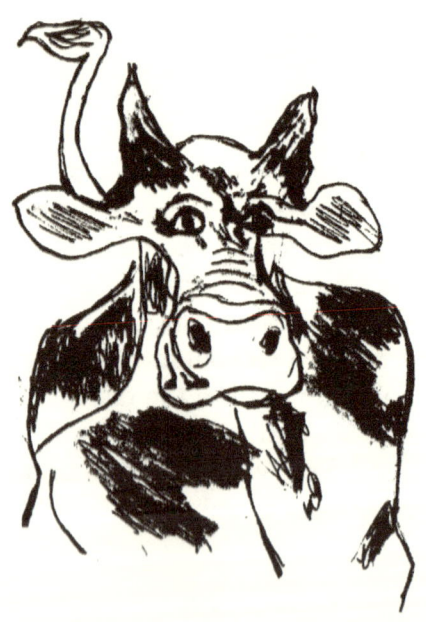

milk instead of one of those huge tumblers the convenient stores offer. We will talk later about all that chocolate you put in your milk. Why not replace it with flavorings? This will not cost you an addition to your waistline.

Watch your serving size. Why measure what you eat? It is very important to realize the quantity of what you eat beforehand. I use little custard dishes and fill them in the morning so I will know the quantities I am partaking of. It is so easy to open the fridge door, eyeball everything and grab a quick bite while standing in front of it.

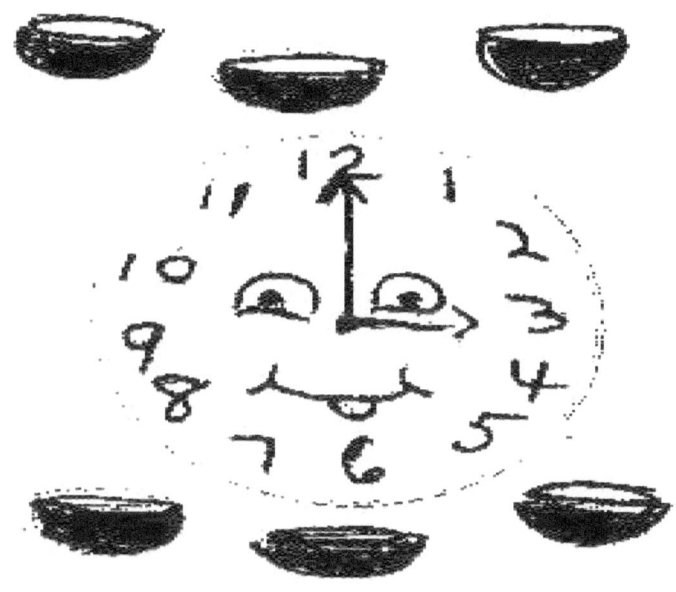

In order to lose weight or maintain your desired weight, of course we must break these habits and continue on filling up our little custard dishes in the a.m.(until we learn moderation), and reserving a shelf in the fridge for just myself, I will be getting a better idea of what and how much I am eating every day.

I believe my biggest problem is when my children and grandchildren are visiting. I have a tendency to make one of those Grand Slam breakfasts and I still have that desire to cook pies, cakes, desserts and everything they like and guess what, I join them! Holiday cooking is so crucial that I go to a good cookbook that makes me aware of making everything lighter. Once you get in the habit of cooking lighter, even Grandmother's old recipes will have to be altered . . . Think change, think slimmer, every time you eat. Whenever I feel the urge rising up in me to eat my mother's famous dish of Pig's Feet and Greens, I think of a nice tossed salad instead. Always have that area of your brain thinking lighter when offered the old method. It's a new day, it's a new day of the Lord, it's a day of joy and gladness, a victory to be won.! Train your mind to watch your serving size. "THINK LIGHT."

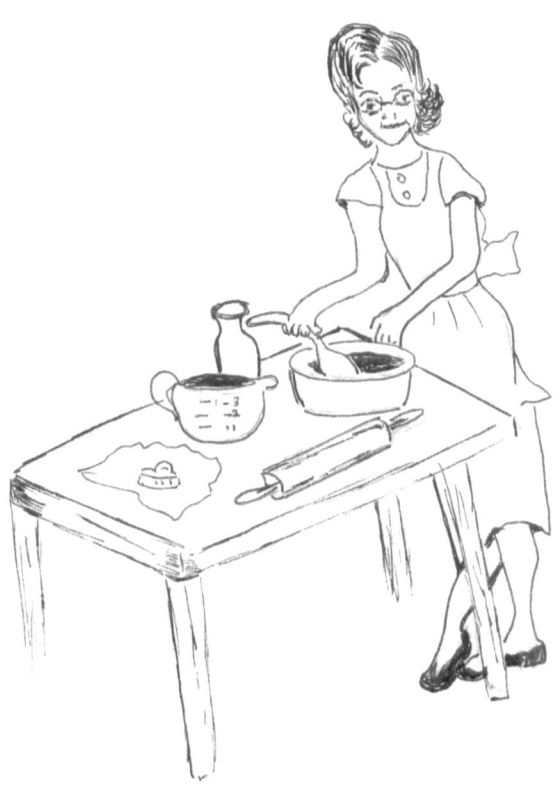

Let's see what else is on the top shelf—condiments, juices. Yes, isn't apple juice and orange juice a great way to get started for the day? Remember, we are only looking at fat right now and these two are 0 grams. That's good! Always drink out of a six ounce glass. You will be surprised how much better you feel when you reduce the amount you drink and eat. When the urge comes to guzzle more, rinse your glass, put it in the dishwasher and say, "NO." "No" isn't such a bad word and we teach it to babies and fail to employ it in our adult lives. Discipline should be a daily word in our vocabulary, as well as bringing our mind into subjection to the will of God, which will cause us to rise up and be the man or woman He wants us to be.

"Casting down arguments and every high thing that exalts itself against the knowledge of God, bringing every thought into captivity to the obedience of Christ." <u>II Corinthians 10:5</u>

I just want you to take your eyes away from the refrigerator for a moment and tell you that without Jesus in my life I could never accomplish anything and I wouldn't even start to pay attention to alternatives or my eating habits. Oddly, without our first cup of coffee, we suddenly realize even our brain is lacking something. I must, yes, you heard me right, have my cup of high test before I can think! (Let's break for a moment so I can go put my coffee on!) We actually think a cup of coffee is the answer for triggering our brain into action.

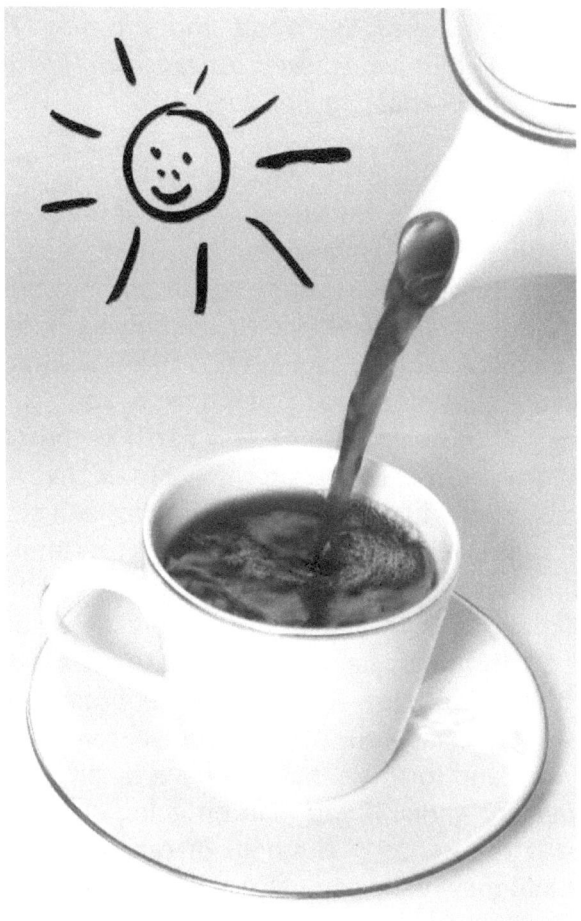

Every time I flick the TV on it's about a new way to lose weight. "Lose 10 lbs" in one week and people buy into this and spend unnecessary dollars on all kinds of junk. If you lose weight fast, you will not keep it off. August 2005 to August 2006, I lost thirty pounds by following the common sense approach I have incorporated in this book. By the way, I have kept this weight off, except for 4-5 pounds and when I see the scale flying upward, I put my goody two shoes on and immediately return to home base. That is a five year plan accomplishment.

"For God so loved the world, that He gave His only Begotten Son, that whosoever believes on Him will not perish but have everlasting life." John 3:16

Let's contemplate on what we ate yesterday. It was Sunday and I drank a shake for breakfast, went out to dinner with some friends after church and did not count the cost and ate all the things I shouldn't have, like fried this, creamed that, heavy sauces etc. You know what I mean 'cause you are just as human as I am. Now don't get a guilt trip! After all, shouldn't we be less harsh on ourselves at least one day a week? But an alternative to this heavy eating on Sunday, would be to get up on Monday, and start your day with coffee, juice and let your stomach rest until at least noon. Since I consumed so much food yesterday, I am going to start my meal with a glass of water (you can use an 8 oz glass for this one); I am going to make myself a tossed salad with good stuff like adding tomatoes, broccoli, carrots, cauliflower, radishes, celery and of course, romaine lettuce and spinach and for me, I have to have a daily onion and fresh elephant garlic. If you plan on going out that night, omit the latter. Honestly, the dogs or cats at home are so tolerant and they really don't care if I eat garlic or onions!

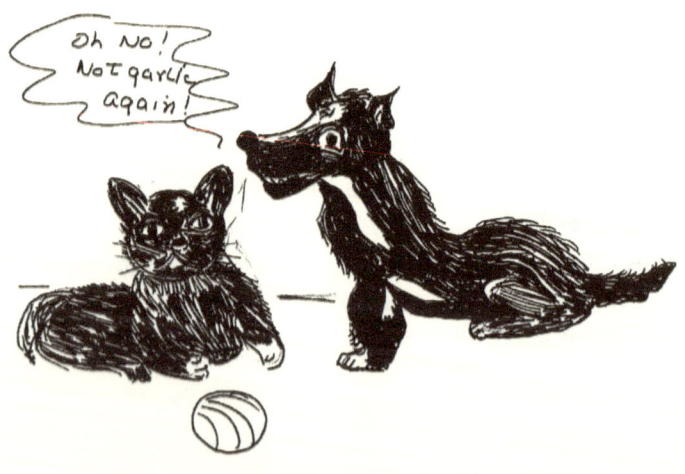

Many times we wake up tired, not really knowing the cause. We stop before we go shopping at the market place and weigh ourselves. Immediately we are overwhelmed that the scale has jumped two pounds since yesterday. Actually, we are composed of 75% water and there is bound to be an increase at times in our weight without gaining weight. But it scares us, it annihilates our desire to lose weight if we are obese. Refrain from weighing yourself each day, check the tightness of your pants when you button up. It is a better gauge to weight gain.

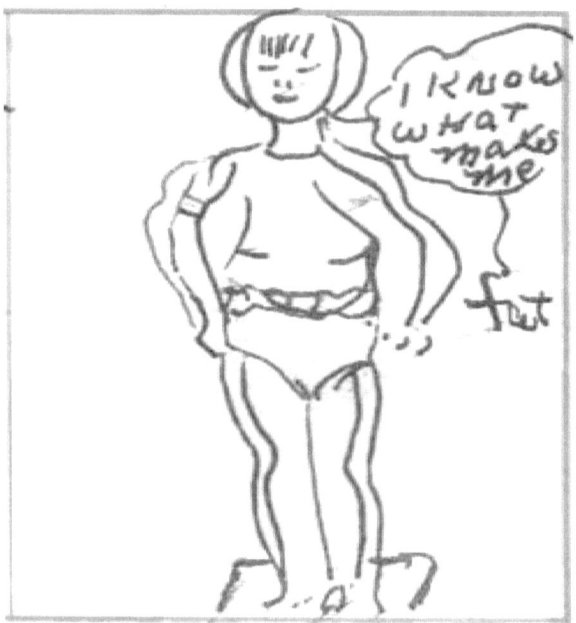

Breakfast should consist of four egg whites with one yolk. Sometimes I use the yolks for puddings or pound cake. How about one of these custard cups holding hot oatmeal, sprinkled with wheat germ or your favorite kind of cereal? Kashi is a good choice. Take charge in your life with using less sugar, salt and change your taste buds to accept a little less sweetness. Delight in changing your taste buds! After all, aren't we sweet enough just as we are? Ahem. Convince yourself of that, please. Are you getting the picture? Smaller quantities and yes, I understand men do consume more calories than women, so perhaps their custard dishes can be the size of a cereal bowl. By using these custard dishes, it makes me more aware of the quantity I eat. Use Smaller glasses . . .

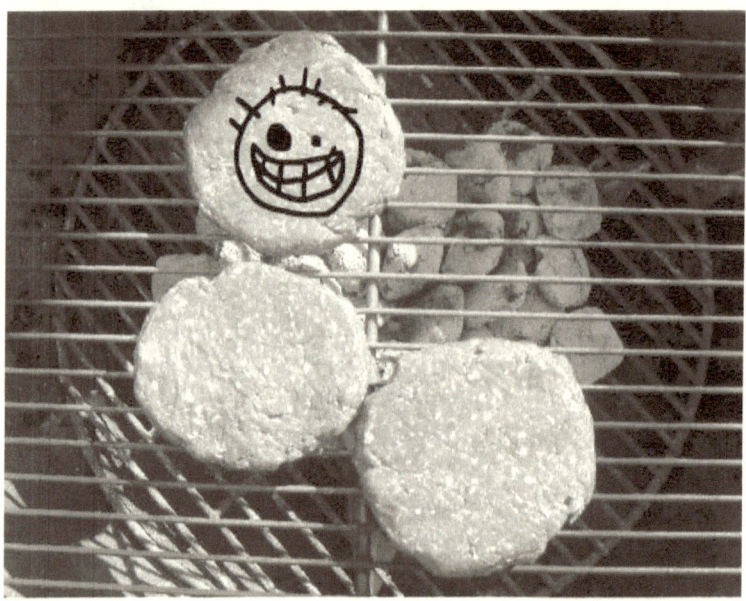

Have you ever ground up a piece of meat? Realize the volume of that triples in size and you are actually putting that much in your stomach at one clip! Once you get use to eating less and more often, you are going to keep a balance.

In order to lose weight or maintain desired weight, we must break these habits and by filling up my little dishes in the a.m. and reserving a shelf in the fridge for just yourself, you will be getting a better idea of what and how much you are eating each day.

I teach my piano students the basics and that is all you need to do with food. Remember there is no short step for losing weight; it takes working at it and it will not happen overnight. You didn't gain 80 pounds over night, nor will it leave any faster than you gained it. Sometimes tho, I do feel I gain faster! Why do we think we have to look like a Barbie doll in order to be happy? We act like the aging process is something to be avoided. It's going to happen folks!

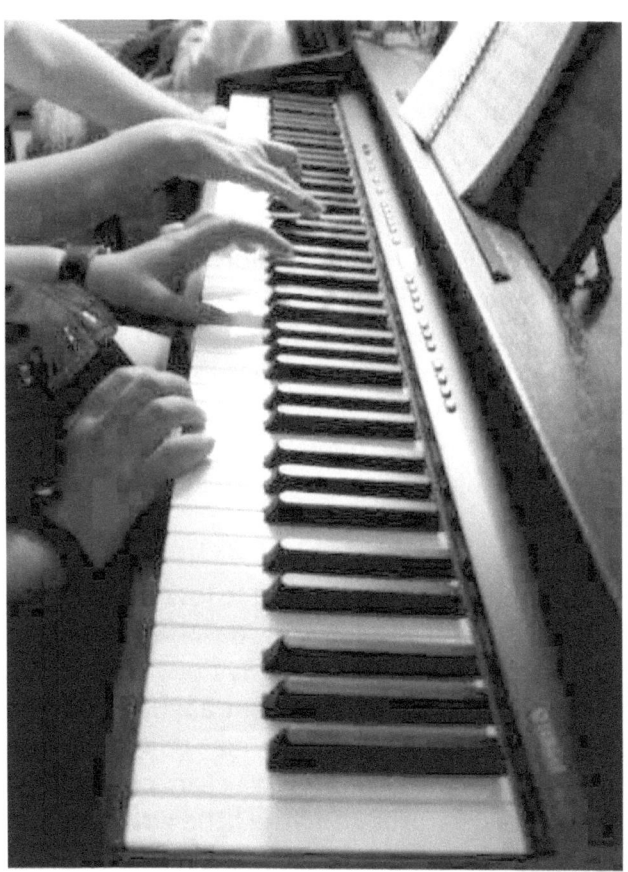

Now I want to tell you something about timing. Upon arising, water, beverage (no sodas or carbonated drinks) and juice, usually orange juice, but it can be tomato or apple juice and I do not begin eating for the day until noon or around that time. If you will make it a way of life and eat a tossed salad every day around noon and make it a chef's salad with low fat turkey or chicken slices and perhaps some feta cheese for flavor and use low fat dressings, along with crackers or a couple slices of bread, rinsed down with either water or hot tea (no iced tea with sugar) or drink iced tea with lemon, you are now initiating a healthy way of life. Hmmmm . . . . where is the protein? I keep hard boiled eggs ready so I can remove the whites and chop them up in my salad (four egg whites, and one egg yolk. "I just don't like to waste, but remember, if you eat the yolks, which contain fat, they will go to waist." I employ this practice, beginning with breakfast, when I'm tempted to eat a grand slam breakfast.

Well, half a day has gone by, I am not starving; in fact I feel rather satisfied. Around 3 o'clock I find myself looking for something to eat. Drink your water first and then enjoy some grapes, apple or any fresh fruit. Try to stay away from canned fruit. However, I do keep a supply of applesauce in the little containers or yogurt for a moment of rewarding myself with something in between. Notice, the amounts are small and I only use one small container.

Dinner time has arrived! I used to love my Mother's raw fried potatoes, fried chicken, pot roasts, soups, dumplings and I still do! But I don't need it! My body sometimes cries out for it and I indulge (don't count anything on Sunday); just be faithful Monday thru Saturday. If I go to a buffet on Sunday I eat anything I like. That way I am preparing myself for Monday thru Saturday and the little girl in me who still doesn't want to say "no" gets a break from the discipline of the week. Actually, you won't gain weight from being naughty one day a week. Another thing, eventually, you won't desire those sweets like you use to. Good eating habits will eliminate your desire for the foods you don't need in your system. When I go to a buffet, even though I have a desire for things I didn't eat all week, I fill my first plate up with toss salad, veggies and anything on the salad bar, accompanied with hot tea, and by the time I get around to eating fried chicken, etc., the amounts I take are much smaller than if I had grabbed that kind of food first. It still pays to keep your healthy way of living going at all times.

Back to the top shelf of the fridge—mayonnaise, salad dressing, dressings for those low calorie lettuce leafs, can all add up to an astonishing amount of fat. Again, I personally do not like fat-free anything and I use reduced fat or light. Yuck! I just realized I have a jar of mayonnaise that is 7.5 grams of fat! Chuck it in the garbage because if you put it in your tummy, it is going to add inches and it will be settling around your middle.

Well, I really got off on a tangent and left the refrigerator door open while typing, so that gives me an opportunity to clean it out this Monday morning and remove all the undesirables that are in it. It is beyond me why I put all those leftovers back in there. Some get pushed to the back and have fuzzy fur growing on them. Hmmm . . . here's some carrots I cooked yesterday. I never fully cook them so they have a little crunch to them. I guess it would be alright to eat these for a snack this morning with a dash of honey. (Actually any dashes you add won't make you fat, because there is not enough calories in a dash to warrant that.) So enjoy the taste of honey on your carrots, which are a good source of beta carotene as well as a shot of Vitamin A. And the honey? Well, honey, it might give you a shot of energy. If you don't like carrots, try celery, if you don't like celery, try? By the way, while I'm on this kick, fix a tray of raw veggies for the day, as well as a fruit platter. If you have grandchildren, they will like peanut butter in the celery sticks and you can use low fat cream cheese as well. In the middle of your dish, put some pistachios on that tray and be sure to have raw carrot sticks and fruit. Stop giving them pastry snacks etc.

Getting back to the fridge again—yes, we are still on the top shelf; make your own dips so you know what is in them; otherwise you could be filling up your stomach with too much fat for the day. I know, they have low fat ones, but for the amount they give you, you could buy a whole 16 oz container of low fat sour cream and add a package of onion mix, ranch mix, etc., and know what you are eating. Sometimes I feel we do not know what we are partaking of and that is when we add to the rim of the tire already around our waist.

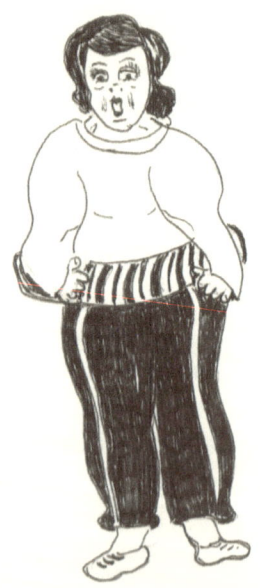

"I can do all things through Christ who strengthens me."
Philippians 4:13

An apple a day keeps the doctor away. How true! My sister-in-law couldn't stand to hear her husband munching on apples and actually he had to eat them, of all places, in the bathroom! I trust you are more tolerant of your mate. Apples contain nutrients that give us energy plus pectin that is a natural stomach and bowel protector. If you get a bout with diarrhea, the pectin from apples will restore your acid levels. All the things He made for us without taking a chemical pill from the doctor!

"All things were made through Him and withouth Him nothing was made that was made." *John 1:3*

Apples have been around a long time, in fact since the Stone Age. By the Fourth Century A.D., the Romans could list 37 different varieties of apples. There are 7,000 varieties in the United States alone. I was raised in New York State, where apples of all kinds were part of our daily diet. Mmmm . . . Mom's homemade apple pie was always our favorite. *(Yes, I make pies, but I do not use lard from ole porky).* I just want to say that apples are coated with wax. Before eating, try to wash off the wax by scrubbing the fruit lightly with a vegetable brush under hot, soapy water. Yes, you heard me right—hot, soapy water! Here is a good tip—apples produce a gas, *Ethylene*, which hastens ripening; placing an apple in a bag with unripe bananas, will soon result in ripe bananas. Don't place apples in a bowl near other ripened fruits, as they will become overripe. By the way, another good tip—place a cut apple in your cookie jar. It keeps them soft. Apples contain potassium and vitamin A, but an even better benefit is Fiber. All senior citizens take note of that! Oh yes, a medium-sized apple has only 80 calories.

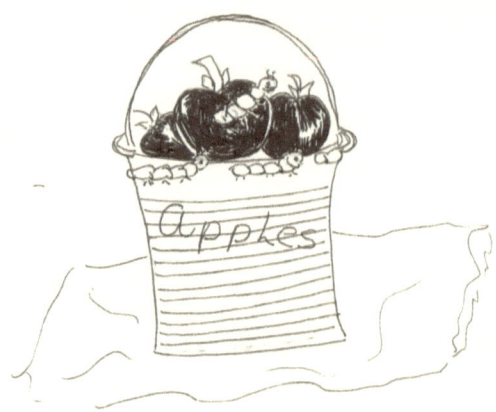

The Holy Spirit that dwells within me is my teacher, my guide, my comforter, and when He tells me what to ingest and what not to, I listen! Putting God's spiritual food first in the morning, before your feet hit the floor, will give you the strength you will need to fight the desire for wrong eating, wrong living. Isn't God good? HE IS, ALL THE TIME!

However, when He the Spirit of Truth has come, He will guide you into all truths. John 16:13

By now you are probably loathing going back to your refrigerator. Well, open the door and let's resume cleaning. I want to be a person that is helping others, not a drudge. There is a possibility that you have other delights on your first shelf and if you do, you can tell by the fat content in them, whether to trash or not. Remember nothing over 2.5 fat content will enter thy mouth!

I just glanced over at my table—Glory be to God! Get rid of that salt shaker on your table. It is more habit than flavor when you douse more salt on your food. I am seeing senior citizens walking around with swollen ankles due to too much salt in their diet. Now most people say, *"Oh, its not the salt that's causing that, I have . . . . and they give you a list of their ailments."* Well, think about it, perhaps your ailments came from that salt shaker. No two ways about it, we really know how to make excuses for everything and as we approach middle age we are so set in our ways that it is mind boggling . . . Don't be fooled by sea salt; there is no proven evidence that it is better for you than salt from the ground. Another money-making idea, many condiments that don't say "salt" such as soy sauce, tamari, hydrolyzed vegetable protein, pickled veggies, cured meats, bouillon cubes, contain high proportions of sodium.

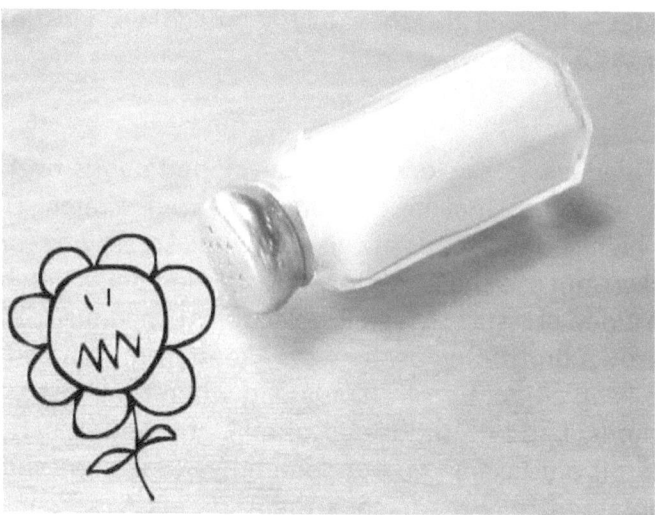

"For since the creation of the world, His invisible attributes, His eternal power and divine nature, have been clearly seen, being understood through what has been made, so that they are without excuse." Romans 1:20

I just cooked a medley of vegetables and while I was typing, I overcooked them all! I am not going to toss them out and the very first thought that came to my mind was, I can lavish a quarter stick of margarine on it, add salt and pepper and store in the refrigerator for my next two main meals. I gently removed the pan from the stove, drained it and said "NO" to butter and salt. Instead, for flavor I will add some roasted dried garlic and pepper. Your taste buds will be delighted and hopefully, you won't overcook your veggies. Think about all those nutrients going down the drain. I believe I will add some carrots and veggies to my food processor and throw a handful or two on my overcooked veggies—that will give them a little crunch! Ok, I just heard your taste buds saying, "NO."

Needless to say, one of my developed habits over the years is always making chicken soup from scratch. Don't buy high sodium soups at the store. It is so easy to cook a chicken and use the broth for soup. Remember, if you have high blood pressure, it is well worth taking the time to make your own broth. One of the ways I keep from using butter, is to keep chicken broth handy and when I make mashed potatoes, I add broth instead of milk and butter. I know I am a bit old fashioned, but sometimes I take ten pounds of potatoes, peel them, cook them up, mash, season and if you put them in small containers or plastic bags you can just defrost that day for dinner and lo and behold, I have spent much less money than from buying them at the store. However, I have found that if you do freeze them, use milk

(1%) instead of chicken broth, because they do not freeze well with chicken broth. By the way, any chicken broth I keep, I allow it to stand overnight in the fridge so I can skim the saturated fat off the top. You do not need that extra fat. (And please don't give it to your pets, as they will develop pancreatitis.)

Here are some eggs, leftover pancakes, toss it; piecrust let me see what the fat content on this one is. Fantastic! Only 1.5 grams of fat, and now, what am I going to fill this pie crust with? I'll let you know further down in this book as I am not ready to start cooking yet today. If it's cream cheese, it won't be the one I have in the fridge as there is 7.5 grams of fat in one little block. I'm tossing that one too. You can save a heap of money by reading the labels while you are shopping. But remember, if it says 7.5 grams toss it, better to waste than to go to waist. (I already said that, didn't I?) I'm always repeating myself. There is something about age that causes that, I think. Some of my children live with me and occasionally do not pay attention to fat content or labels.

Certainly there are enough spices in this country to satisfy our cravings. In fact, I just ate my lunch, a tossed salad with broccoli, romaine lettuce, cauliflower, tomatoes, onion, elephant garlics (I always use the elephant kind 'cause it is not as strong as regular garlic), carrots, a 6 oz glass of 1% milk, soy milk or almond—your choice! (I need that calcium and so do you), a tablespoon of honey mustard on my salad and here is a good tip if you have esophagus problems—you are probably right now saying you can't eat tossed salad due to the roughage effect in your throat—I get my food processor out and grind it up, Yes, even the lettuce, and I am getting the same benefit as someone who chomps each piece for five minutes or if you are like my children, they can inhale their food in one breath and I'm sitting there thirty minutes later eating by myself. And by the way, I chopped up four cooked egg whites and one egg yolk; added it to my salad and gave the yolks to my dog, Daisy. She looked at them rather funny, but finally ate them. I hope I am not giving my dog high cholesterol!

My lunch was very satisfying and I am now eyeing the clock—goodness gracious! I really have a messed up time clock today—I am actually eating my lunch at 2:30! These are some red flags that you need to heed. Try to get a regular time to eat each day and that is going to take some more discipline. With the busy lives we lead these days, I'm fluffing this one off 'cause yesterday was Sunday and I ate everything I shouldn't have, so perhaps the length of time that I actually put something in my stomach was a quieting down rest on my heart and organs.

Recently, I was sitting in a restaurant and the guy next to me ordered ribs. Well, let me tell you, it was "all you can eat" day and he had a stack of bones on his plate as high as Mt. Everest. My thought was, *"He must have consumed two pounds of meat, not counting the baked potato, beans, etc., that he had eaten."* Overeating or overtaxing our organs will cause some big troubles up ahead. Because he, like anyone else, will end up with bypass surgery, kidney stones, liver problems, pancreatic failure? Just a little planning before you go to a restaurant will help you curb that "Overeating" attack.

Another restaurant had a sign up, *"All the crabs you can eat for $39.95 and please do not share with your neighbor."*

Give me a break guys, what on earth do you think the size of my stomach is? Yes, again I want you to know, it is no larger than your fist and if you have filled it so full, you are distressing all your internal organs. Wake up America and live! (The only reason I say America is 'cause I live here).

By now everything in my refrigerator must be soggy and ready for the garbage can, 'cause I left it open so I wouldn't forget to clean it (I really don't advise you to do this), but I want you to get a picture of what you need to do and what you need to throw out.

Let's go to shelf Number 2—Let me see what I have here that needs to be tossed. Oh, by the way, I usually put a label on leftovers, the date and what they are. Come on, sometimes I can look at something and not know what it is. One good clue, besides the label, is to smell it, and that is one of my top tips—smell it. "When in doubt, throw it out." Don't become such a penny pincher that you will eat something possibly spoiled to save a nickel. The doctor's bill would be several hundred times that nickel Ok, yes we have arrived at shelf 2. Hmmm . . . . let me see—Gosh, I hope your fridge doesn't look like mine! I mean, how did this happen? Such a variety of things, I don't know what to do with them. Actually, I can give myself a brownie point 'cause I always store everything in plastic containers or plastic bags. Never leave anything open to the air. It not only makes your refrigerator smell bad, but I personally think it can pick up on bacteria, (oh yes, its floating everywhere,) plus get that yucky fridge smell. While I'm thinking about it, put some baking soda in a small cup or buy a fridge soda box, place on shelf 3 way in the back, out of sight. It cuts down on the odor of food, as well as any leftovers that might have been pushed to the back. I really shouldn't tell on myself, but actually this could happen to anyone—it's a disgusting thought though and I hesitated whether I should tell you or not, 'cause you might not want to eat at my house ever again. Well, I am going to tell on myself. Somehow or another, a fly flew in my refrigerator and when I went to get some eggs for breakfast, there he was, flat on his back dead as a doornail. Poor guy froze to death. I don't know why I had to say this, but I did and I'm glad. Actually, you will be happy to know I scrubbed that spot where he laid. Safety first for all things.

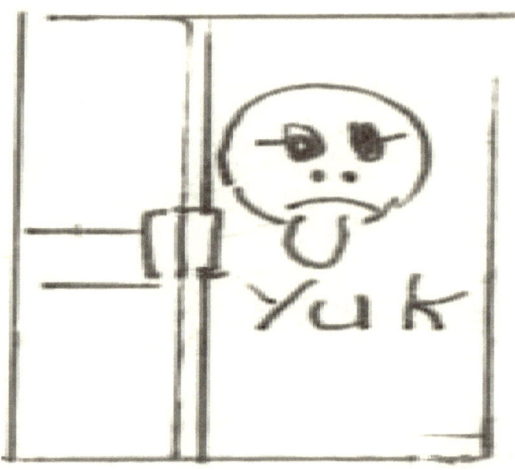

No wonder I did not shut the fridge door! It would hardly close! I have so many things on shelf 2! Spaghetti sauce, cooked angel hair spaghetti, (that's about the only kind we like); a large tub of margarine, (the one without trans fat); cut up honeydew melon, chicken soup, (this one you really want to watch for spoilage as it shouldn't be kept longer than a couple of days in the fridge.)

I definitely am going to have to use up those mixed veggies I started unthawing the other night—guess they will take their place in the chicken soup I am making. Do not use any skin of the chicken and preferably use the white meat instead of the dark, as the dark contains more fat and cholesterol.

Shelf 2 is looking better now that I tossed most of it out and the dibs and dabs in jars like catsup, horseradish and the ginger mix which shocked me when I read that it had 7.5 grams of fat in it! Is 7.5 a famous number or something? Maybe I ought to start playing the lotto and use 7 and 5. Sometimes I wonder who makes up all these rules and regulations, not only on food, but my tax return as well. God never said we couldn't have a sense of humor and I trust you know that if I sound sarcastic once in awhile, it's because truly I don't know all the answers, but am forever seeking His Knowledge on whatever is involved with my life. Are you getting the picture?

"Wise people store up knowledge, but the mouth of the foolish is near destruction. Proverbs 10:14"

I am really too tired to do shelf 3 right now and would rather give you some more insight and facts at the present moment. I hope you are enjoying this household trip with me.

I don't know about you, but I can only speak from experience. I think we become like rabbits and think we have to nibble all the time on something. If we don't nibble, then we smoke a cigarette, (not me though, I don't smoke) and some people chew on a toothpick. As adults we still need pacifiers. It's like that urging or craving for something to satisfy our inner being that never leaves us. To tell you the truth, I am a nibbler. One of the ways I have overcome eating all the time and still continue grazing is to have a bowl of raw veggies chopped up, a pan of rice, (sorry I don't like brown rice, yes I know it's better for us, but I like white rice); mix your veggies with the rice, add a dash of roasted garlic or whatever spice you like, (I use a lot of fresh ginger); vinaigrette, in a moderate amount; keep this mixture on eye level in the refrigerator and when you think you need a steak, eat a couple of tablespoons. You will find that it not only satisfies but it also calms a bit of a desire for sweets, ice cream etc., Unusual cravings flee!

I don't expect you to try everything I say in this book, but I do know that it works for me. It does something to our metabolism and your hunger pains and desires will leave. Now I am speaking explicitly to people who want to lose weight or need to lose weight. In no way do I ever want you to be on a diet, as diets don't cut it and when you return to your old eating habits, the fat comes right back on. I call it the Yo-Yo Syndrome. A Golden Nugget Way of Life is to use the wisdom God has given us and stay on that Highway to Heaven by eating healthy and being the person He wants you to be.

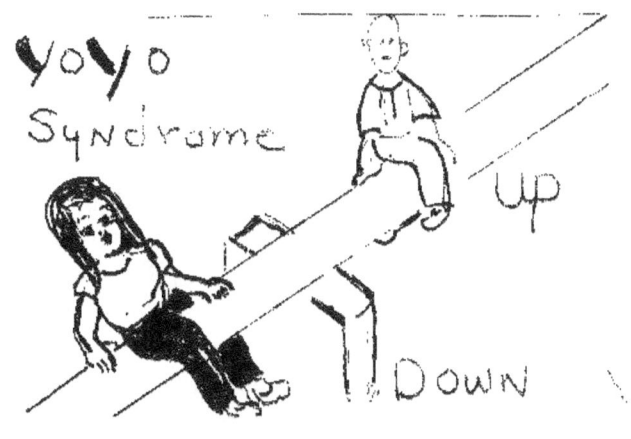

"You are the light of the world. A city that is set on a hill cannot be hidden. Nor do they light a lamp and put it under a basket, but on a lampstand and it gives light to all who are in the house." Matthew 5:14

Speaking about a bushel basket, buy fruits and fresh veggies in quantities; Take those specked bananas and make banana bread; Oh yes, there is bound to be some spoilage, but the benefits of keeping grapes, kiwis, bananas, apples, etc., in a bowl will help you acquire good eating habits and I find my children and grandchildren always partake of whatever I have on the counter. One good tip—if strawberries are not eaten up fast enough, I wash them and place them in a container in the freezer for shakes; likewise blueberries and bananas (don't throw that banana out if it is specked with brown; freeze it also, for shakes). Why buy canned green beans, carrots, etc. when you can go to the market and get fresh veggies? They are so much more flavorful and appealing to the eye, as well as to the stomach. I love to can, however, and at the end of the week I make soups of all kinds with leftover vegetables, (not the ones with the fur on them); meats, poultry, etc., and usually bring my canner out and use these soups all during the year.

Okay, lets get back to Shelf 3 in my fridge—I'm afraid to look! Actually, shelf 3 looks the best, but odd, how fresh hamburger got on that shelf instead of in the meat tray. (We have many hands going in and out of my fridge but I am usually the worst enemy and I find myself hastily sometimes putting things away and forgetting about them). At the time there seemed to be a rhyme and reason for my reasoning, but as time went by and other things were shoved in the refrigerator, the meat got pushed to the back and I don't know how old it is, so out it goes in the garbage can! Here's a can of condensed milk. I actually have a craving for such sweet stuff, so that is going out also. Anything I can't overcome the temptation for, it is now out of my fridge. Well, the bottom trays contain mostly things like potatoes, celery, squash and all good earthly things, so I don't have to say a lot about the last two drawers. Sometimes though, I hide things from the children, like my good yogurt and need to keep track of such odds and ends. There are times though when I have reached for something and found dead, dead, lettuce, but on the whole I keep pretty good tabs on fresh fruits and veggies.

Remember that old song by Carmen Miranda? *"I'm Chiquita Banana and I come to say, bananas they must ripen in a certain way. When they are flecked with brown and have a golden hue, bananas are so good and they are good for you!"* But remember; never put the banana in the refrigerator.

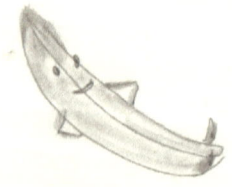

Sometimes we hold onto things we have been taught down thru the years by our parents. We did not have refrigeration in the 30's, with the exception of a block of ice in our "ice box" or snow on the outside window sill to keep our milk cold.

One thing I didn't adhere to was my mother giving us black strap molasses every Spring to spruce up the iron in our blood; although I did like her Molasses Cookies.

Honestly, I can sure fly off the original subject of losing weight and eating healthy, including all the golden nuggets I have given you; but Moms do make memories. And even though my Mother never took any courses on what was good for us, she was right on target and we lived off the huge garden my Dad planted every Spring. The proof is in the pudding, as my Mother would say and I can honestly say that none of us were ever overweight. By the way, we lived on homemade bread, cookies, beef, pork and all the things they say you shouldn't eat today. What was the difference? Our lifestyle—we were always playing outside after school in the snow banks, sledding, skating, never in the house until suppertime. Today's children are doing their homework and then sitting in front of the Nintendo or TV until bedtime. I can't say that is true for all children, but wherever I go, I find them peering into a game boy or seated in front of the TV. As parents, you need to realize that you should have control of that and act accordingly. Our nation is producing obese children like never before!

Whatever happened to children working and planting a garden, picking strawberries etc? There are so many outdoor sports they should be participating in. I am always happy to see them playing ball or gymnastics but I really believe this has become a minority in our country.

Now that my refrigerator is back to normal and is clean, I want to open the cupboard doors. Swing wide open and let's see what we need to get rid of in here. Really, I am trying to become the person God wants me to be, so all the junk in here is going to have to go! I see lots of sugar, assorted canned goods that have been in there forever; ramen noodles, macaroni and cheese (that has to stay 'cause my grandchildren love it), but I won't eat it and really it is not a temptation for me. Jell-O—now that is a good dessert. We should make some of that up every day, the kind without all the sugar, of course. I do believe that children need more starch than we do as adults, so granted, I give in to some of their desires. I hope I am not promoting bad habits down the road. I guess the canned goods, like beets, etc., can stay 'cause there are times when you will be in a pinch for a vegetable and that will come in handy. But don't make it a habit to replace canned goods for fresh ones.

Just by emptying my fridge and cupboards of all undesirables and know that I am going to look at the labels before I purchase anything, makes me feel a couple pounds lighter already! Are you getting the picture? It is not difficult to lose weight and we must give up our alibis for being fat. So many think it's their thyroid, (when in actuality it is their eating habits). If someone says to you, "I can't lose weight," it is an alibi. They need to take a hard look at themselves and be honest and I think any of us who have a handle on nutrition, *"Know what makes us fat."* I know I do and I have often said, *"Try it, you might like it"* and for the next twelve weeks and the rest of my life I plan on incorporating good eating habits, casting all the old ones away, not overeating, not joining the crowd in their parties where everything is dripping with fat.

"I can do all things thru Christ who strengthens me." <u>Philippians 4:13</u>

And do not be conformed to this world, but be transformed by the renewing of your mind that you may prove what is that good and acceptable and perfect will of God. <u>Romans 12:2</u>

Don't overwhelm yourself with days of dieting but rather, enjoy the abundant life God has bestowed on you and if you are a few pounds heavy and you are not happy, incorporate good eating habits and some of the suggestions I have given you and learn to say, "NO." Not everyone is going to be a skinny minny and depending on your bone structure, sometimes you can't go according to those charts for ideal weight. I consider myself 20 pounds overweight, but my doctor says only ten pounds. (That was nice of her). However, if I am not happy with losing only ten pounds then I shall aim for my goal of twenty! Are you getting the picture? By reading this book and following my guidelines, you will lose 30-40 pounds, if that is your goal.

Here are some questions to ask yourself. What do I do when I am not occupied with my job, my mate or my children? Do I use that free time productively or am I in front of the TV 5-6 hours a day with perhaps something to pacify myself before dinner, like sodas, chips and sandwiches? Multiply that by, perhaps Monday thru Friday, and it amounts to around 30-40 hours a week, munching, lazing around with a snack in your hand or you go to pick the children up and stop at McDonalds and have a "bite" to eat or a gooey sundae, accompanied by a fountain drink. I am in no way saying this is everyone's lifestyle, but if this is why you are fat, think about it. Idle time is the devil's workshop and so many times we fall prey to his traps. I really believe one of the main causes of obesity is overeating and eating when we are not hungry. Why do we eat when we are not hungry? Evidently, our body does not need anything or we would hear that giant lion roar coming from our stomach. One way to help this problem would be to think tea, especially green tea, which will cause you to lose 13 pounds a year without trying. (I am taking a TV doctor's word on this one). Drink hot tea, do not add anything to it but the teabag when you feel you have to eat something, and quite frankly you don't have a hunger spot in your stomach. Bringing our minds into subjection to the mind of Christ will cause us to become an overcomer. He, Jesus, wants us to be an overcomer and cross over the finish line some day holding our torch high and finishing the race victoriously.

"Do you not know that those who run in a race all run, but one receives the prize? Run in such a way that you may obtain it. And everyone who competes for the prize is temperate in all things. Now they do it to obtain a perishable crown, but we for an imperishable crown. Therefore, I run thus; not with uncertainty. Thus I fight: not as one who beats the air. But I discipline my body and bring it into subjection, lest, when I have preached to others, I myself should be disqualified." I Corinthians 10:24-27

Okay, we have knocked out the TV set, the idle time, what else could be causing us to be fat? Perhaps our sedentary life style, failing to exercise every day will cause a slump in our thinking, jumping on the scale and being defeated 'cause no weight has come off; looking in the mirror and realizing, "I'm fat." I could almost put a stamp marked, "Guaranteed" weight loss if you will start cutting in half what you usually partake of. Pushing back from the table once you feel that

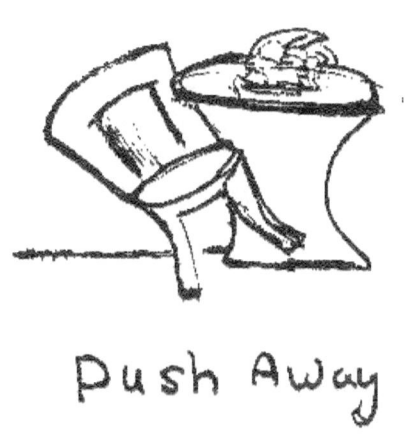

Push Away

full button says, "No more" and not guzzling liquids when you eat, will cause you to rise up and suddenly, you will notice your pants are no longer tight. I don't want to hear your excuses 'cause I know that is what will be coming out of your mouth next. Hold your tongue and realize you are not the only person in the world with this problem. Tell me, what good does it do for you to eat ten pieces of chocolate candy instead of one? Do you feel the other nine are going to make you feel better? That fried chicken isn't so bad if you have only one piece, but if you think you have to have three, at least make sure you are eating boiled chicken without the skin—it will make such a difference in your weight!

I, for one, feel the trend right now is to get rid of this, get rid of that, don't eat carbs and don't eat fat, (Well, we have to have some fat to keep our burners ignited and our evening meal should be a reasonable sized lean hamburger, along with a helping of mashed potatoes or baked potato, minus the butter and sour cream, unless you are going to limit yourself to one tablespoon of each). Again, I cannot stress the importance of eating fresh vegetables, but don't douse them with butter. Drink ice water at dinnertime and allow yourself jello or if it is cake, angel food cake, a high source of protein since it is made with egg whites.

I do not agree with the low carb diet 'cause you are causing your muscles deterioration and they must inhale carbs. If you run or ride a bike you will experience fatigue and muscle cramps due to a lack of carbohydrates in your system. I found this out in one of the medical books I have here in my library.

Back to dinnertime—why do we feel we always have to have meat at dinnertime? It actually takes beef 8-1/2 hours to digest in your system. (I found this in a book written by a doctor in 1910) and if you have an alcoholic drink with your meal, it actually causes your system to overwork another eight hours. Your heart is being overtaxed, which might not show up immediately, but over a period of time the toll it is taking will probably be open heart surgery. Someone might say, "You are listening to ancient history," but actually, whenever I TOOK a glass of wine (past tense), I had the symptoms this doctor described and since, I never have been a drinker. I gave up drink on holidays or whenever I was a social butterfly and those symptoms like rapid heart (an overtaxed heart), and a rush to my brain which I couldn't deal with from one glass of wine; heartburn and the rest, I said all the cards were on the table and I decided "This is not for me." I don't drink pepsi or coke, as they have a bad effect on me, why should I drink wine? I am certainly not telling you to quit anything, that is up to you, but I believe we learn by trial and error and from each other.

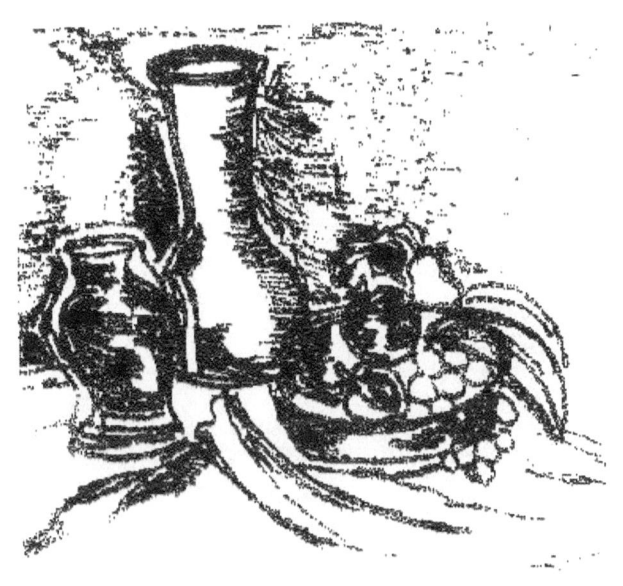

I hope you are enjoying this trip from my fridge and cupboards, to the rest of my house as I plan on being with you for the rest of the week. If you are retired, you probably will identify more with me than someone younger, but we can learn from each other's experiences, regardless of our age. God wants us all to have a teachable spirit and aren't the older ladies and men supposed to help the younger women and men? Children also?

I don't know how I keep getting off the subject of weight and correct eating, which this book is supposedly about and somehow I skipped Tuesday with you. It was an uneventful day and sometimes I get so busy with picking up grandchildren from school that I failed to stay in my house very much that day.

I'm glad we've made it past the kitchen where I spend most of my time, but lets see what is going on during the week in my living room. I find in the early morning, I sit in my comfortable chair with my bible, prop my feet up on the ottoman, and of course, before I do all that I make my coffee, keep a phone close by and drink orange juice or water. Remember to limit your orange juice to six ounces. That doesn't sound too addictive, does it? I never have hunger pains in the mornings anyhow, so it is no biggee for me to just have juice and coffee. So that's not my reason for gaining weight. I guess we can leave that room. Not yet, though.

There are some times when I plop down in the same chair in the afternoon and suddenly I get that urge for chips, dip, ice cream—I want to treat myself. After all, aren't I the main one that cleans this house? How about a few cookies? My brain starts receiving signals from my childhood that tells me I deserve to treat myself. Well, remember, if you want to lose weight, the only time you can treat yourself to anything is on Sunday or whatever day you pick, but it can only be one day per week. So what am I going to replace on this stand next to me? A good alternative would be popcorn, of course, without the butter (an alternative to butter is butter buds, or we enjoy lemon pepper, parmesan cheese), pretzels, a veggie or fruit—apples give us a lift in the afternoon.

Avoid at this time of the day those goodies that are going to create a new gauge around your waistline.

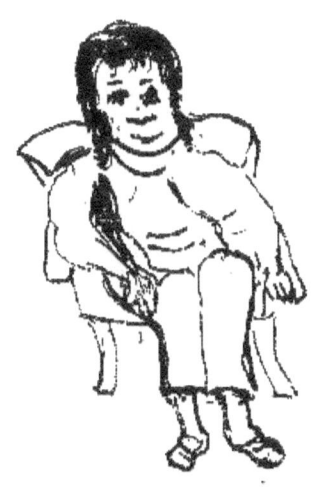

My son and daughter, (we live together), and I, enjoy a homemade shake every day and it is a good energy booster, which we mainly drink in the a.m. It contains either 1% milk, 1 tbs. peanut butter, (the reduced fat kind), a banana, two strawberries, 1/2 apple, a sprinkle of oatmeal, wheat germ, a dash of honey and whatever other fruit is on the counter. Sometimes mango, peaches, and always 1/2 cup plain yogurt, 1/4 cup of crushed ice and the coldness numbs your tummy and guess what, "No Hunger Pains." Believe me, this shake sometimes lasts me until 3 or 4 o'clock and if my time clock is off for the day, I resist eating dinner until around 5:30 pm. Yes, today I took my shake into the living room with me. If you have a diabetic problem, it is better for you to have your shake in the morning.

Start opening your eyes and be aware of what you are putting on your plate. Then, take an inventory of what you have eaten already that day. Instead of eating a complete meal when eating out, eat half and take the rest home. It is very doubtful you will eat the other half 'cause once it has been referred to the refrigerator it has lost its appeal and in my house, Daisy, our dog will eat it. Calorie counting is not such a bad idea. It gives you an assessment of what you can consume the rest of the day. I know by 4-6 pm, I have partaken most of my calorie intake for the day.

I have a cooler in the back of my van, mainly for grandchildren; snacks after school, but I only pick healthy snacks like boiled eggs, fruits, veggies and healthy drinks. For me the healthy drink is water.

I haven't said anything about sleep. How important it is to get eight hours sleep every night. Somehow since I am older, my time clock has switched from 5 to 5 1/2 hours and I am raring to go. An alternative that will help you rest a full eight hours is hot milk and either powdered ginger or one teaspoon of grated fresh ginger, added to the milk. I sleep like a baby. If there is anyone out there who knows what is in ginger that makes one sleep, please let me hear from you. (Truly, I do not know).

Today I ate something I shouldn't have, that is, if I want to lose weight. We must forever be on our toes if this lubber is going to come off. I had fixed a sweet potato—a huge one, with orange juice, brown sugar and cinnamon, smashed it all together and ate it. An alternative here would be to prick a sweet potato, place it in the microwave (wrap in paper towel) and eat it in its natural state. Sometimes I wonder if I can ever overcome my desire to add this and that to everything I eat. Sauces overwhelm me—I love them! Instead of sauces start adding rice vinegar, vinaigrette or a dash of something sweet (honey) if you must have something sweet. Splenda is a very good outlet for that, although I do not care for artificial sweeteners and just recently I read that they can be a cause of cancer. A teaspoon of sugar only has 17 calories and would be a good alternative to dietetic this and that. Over a period of time, reducing things that you are use to will cause you to drop in weight and if you find you can't give something up, start drinking hot tea before your meal or snack time. It is very satisfying. Decaffeinated teas are better. Also, drinking a glass of water before dinner not only aids in digestion, but causes one not to overeat.

Let's talk about that bathroom scale—Yes, I am scurrying you to the bathroom. Never thought I would invite someone into the bathroom—yep, there is that scale that we say is always wrong, five pounds this way or that way, so we adjust the scale to begin on five pounds. We were so good yesterday that we are going to jump out of bed and race to the bathroom to weigh ourselves to see how much we lost. How downright discouraging. It says I gained three pounds. Well, that way of life is not for me and we return to our old eating habits. Instead of staying steadfast we become discouraged and defeated. I only weigh myself once a month and if there is a significant change in my weight, then I must sit down and count the costs. Where did I fail with this new regime? Perhaps it isn't for me? Did I consistently cheat all month, making alibis? Am I remaining in my old way of life?

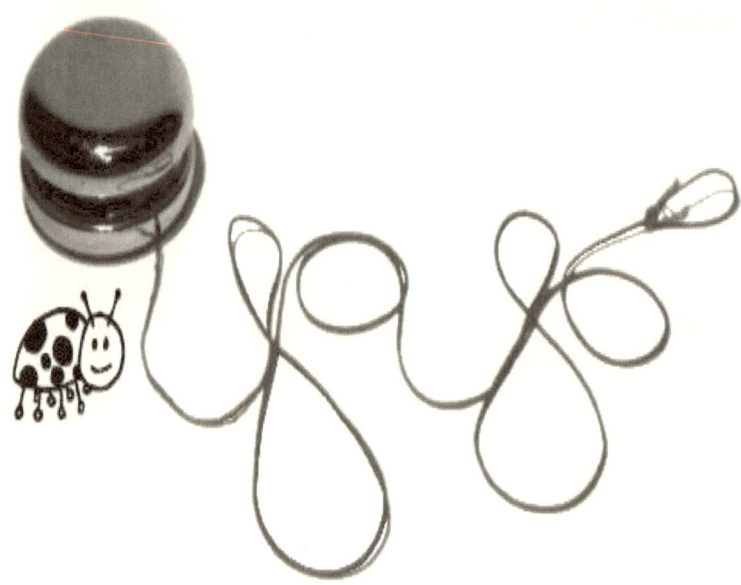

Jesus said we are transformed by the renewing of our minds and that means daily. If you think you can be a Yoyo bouncing up and down, that tells me you haven't changed a thing in your life. Twelve weeks of discipline will start you on the right path and you will see a weight loss if you continue on your way of life, instead of making excuses. I find it is better not to relate to the world what you are trying to do, 'cause they will batter you when you go to restaurants and the like and start watching everything you are eating. Best, that you remain silent and eventually they are going to be saying, "Are you losing weight?" You really look good!" And remember the story of my sweet potato—just because I failed doesn't mean I can't get up and renew my mind and start over. Don't let one sweet potato cause you to call it quits and throw in the towel.

Actually, my bedroom contains every book that was ever written, weights, torso track, computer, sewing machine, fax machine, tv. Since it is in a handy place on the wall facing my bed, it caused me never want to get up and make my bed. A good alternative are Christian stations and I have learned so much about nutrition through our friends, Seventh Day Adventists' doctors. Why do we feel we have to belong to a certain church group in order to learn from others? Billy Graham is such a model preacher who loves Catholics, Episcopalians and every denomination. He extends his arm of brotherly love to everyone. I'm not sure, but I guess he is a Baptist. Does it really matter? The only time I would draw the line is if someone is not preaching the good news of Jesus Christ. That would make them false.

Speaking of churches, church suppers can really cause you to gain weight if your church has one every week. There is a variety to pick from and instead of picking and choosing, we take a little bit of everything! Very enticing, so before you approach the table, say a little prayer and stay away from anything that looks good, like fried chicken, cakes, pies and all the rest. Speaking about pies, I have had this jar of mincemeat from my trip to Ireland this year, so the other day I made a homemade apple pie and poured the contents of the mincemeat on top of the apples and I am freezing it for a very special day called Christmas. It really didn't appeal to me anyways, but some people do like mincemeat. Imagine the calories—oh well, Christmas Day, one small piece. Eat mostly turkey.

You see how we try to justify everything we eat? It really isn't very nice of me to cause everyone else to get fat.

I just can't seem to get out of the kitchen. Christmas Day will have to be my free day that week so I can taste the mincemeat apple pie. Enough said about that. Back to our tour.

Since I already told you my computer is in the bedroom, I have spent four hours on it writing my story and I plan to bring nothing into this bedroom but a glass of water. Think I'll take a sip. This is a good spot for me to be because I never have the time to think about my stomach. Did you ever notice that we are always wondering what we will eat for dinner when we are eating our breakfast? No wonder our hormones are so active. Our salivary glands never stop dripping, wanting more . . . more . . . .

I have all this exercise equipment in my bedroom, so I think I will stop writing for awhile and lift a few weights and work out on my torso track. If you really expect the pounds to go away, you will have to exercise, as well as eat the right things. I hear people say, "Well, I work all day and get enough exercise that way," but housework or jobs won't cut it. You are going to have to get down and exercise daily. I have a daughter who has a trainer and the results of her exercising, along with eating properly has brought about her desired weight loss—but she had to be consistent and do it every day.

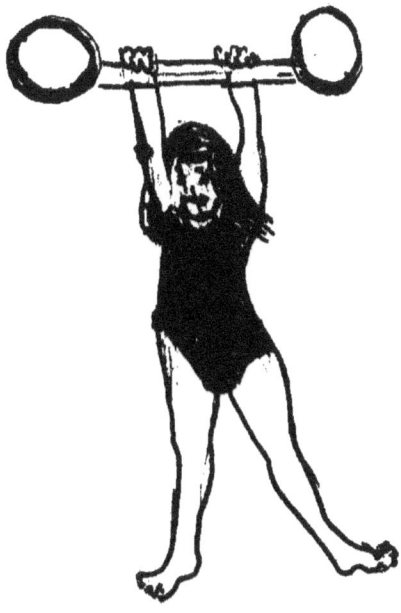

No excuses! And in order for her to maintain her changed way of life, she is going to have to put into practice daily what she has learned, not a diet to keep her in good condition, but a way of life.

I place two five pound weights by my table and when I sit down I do twelve reps, occasionally getting up and doing lower abs. If you place your weights near where you are sitting you are more likely to use them than if they are hid in a closet. Keep a radio handy and play a CD, spend some time dancing every day. It is a wonderful way to burn calories and I cannot tell you how much enjoyment it gives me.

Exercise has so many benefits. It counters heart disease and stroke by lowering serum cholesterol levels and blood pressure and by helping the heart to pump more blood with less effort. It strengthens muscle tone in the legs, and exercise can prevent and sometimes reverse the symptoms of varicose veins. Your blood sugar levels will improve—exercise helps to lower blood sugar. This effect helps to counter diabetes. Exercise strengthens your bones and prevents the loss of calcium that weakens bones as people age. Your joints aching? Exercise helps to keep joints mobile and if you have arthritis, you will find the benefits immensely helpful. Why not join the YMCA? The prices are good and well worth it.

And what about sleep? Restful sleep comes with exercise! Our unwillingness to try anything new and to use alibis to justify why we can't do something means simply, "I don't want to." Change must come first in your thought patterns.

Again, why do we eat when we aren't hungry? That hunger button should cause us to realize that it is time to eat. A baby cries for food, he sets the alarm off for Mom or Dad to feed him. In fact, a baby is smarter than adults; he refuses to eat if he isn't hungry. So why do we eat when we aren't hungry? Examine yourself, start questioning why, why, why we do what we do? And we can even quote *Shakespeare*—"I pray that I may learn from listening—whether or not I agree with what I hear."

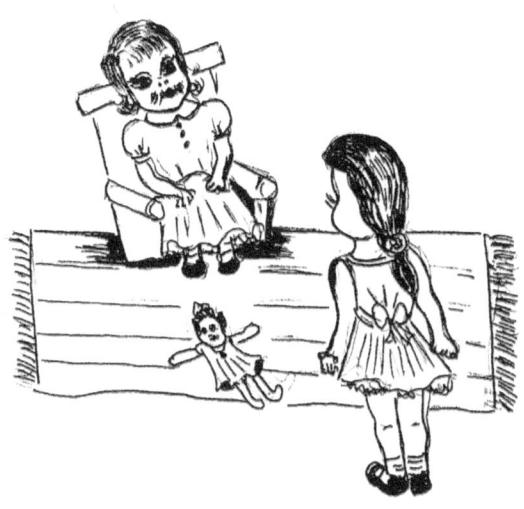

When my children were little, I would do my housework at night because I liked to wake up to a clean house and it gave me more time with my children before I went to work. Without realizing it, I always felt I deserved to reward myself and would drink a couple mugs of hot chocolate and devour a dozen cookies. Then I would go to sleep on that. Luckily, at that point in my life, I was very active and did not gain weight. Were I to do that today, I know the fat would be accumulating around my waist. You may not realize it, but we still think we need to reward ourselves because we have expended ourselves beyond the call of duty. If that is your problem, quit! A bad habit formed needs to be broken before it takes off like a tornado in your life.

Turn your Eyes Upon Jesus and get the focus off food. There are so many things we can do in life, like helping others with their problems and if you look around you will find many people have problems that far exceed your own.

Your thinking processes have to change in order for you to lose weight and when we form a barrier making up all kinds of excuses why we are fat, it is not going to melt away like so many false advertisements promise. If you will follow God's Word and plan for your life, things will change for you. You can desire that change, but if you do not take an action, nothing is going to happen. You will look in the mirror and see a fat stomach, rolls on the side hanging down and even your feet will be spanning over the sides of your sandals. Don't you really care how you look or have you become so defeated that you wallow in self-pity and would rather stay in that state or way of life because it is easier to retreat than go forward? Remember, we are pressing on for the prize of the high calling in Christ Jesus.

I press toward the goal for the prize of the upward call of God in Christ Jesus. Philippians 3:14

One of my biggest problems in losing weight or maintaining weight is the fact that I want instant mashed potato results, "Right now" and I do not want to work at it; I want it handed to me on a silver platter. When that doesn't happen and the scale refuses to jump up and down and shout you lost a few pounds, it grins its ugly face and says you haven't lost anything. But, you say, "I tried all week and nothing happened. What's the use anyhow; I am destined to be fat."

One thing I will pass on to you that has helped me is to study the Word of God. Memorize scriptures, spend more time and money doing the work of God. Be active in your church activities and find friends that will be an encouragement to you and ones that you can also encourage.

Make God the center of your very being. Until we die to self and realize we belong to Him and want to do our very best for Him in all we do, we will continue on the path of self-righteous seeking.

Due to all the fat that is on us, we feel no one could be interested in us. We do find mates regardless. Wouldn't it be nice to get to know who that person is inside that I might plan to live with the rest of my life?

Jesus said to come to Him, just as you are. His arms are wide open, waiting for you to ask Him into your heart. His Agape Love will cause you to think differently and you will start to see others in a different light and a lot of vanity will leave you.

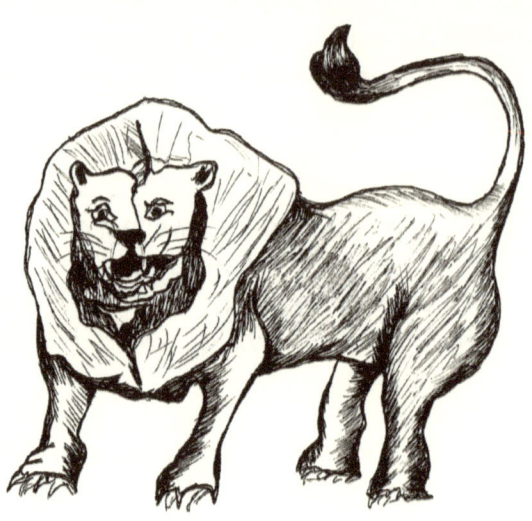

That hungry lion in our stomach announces our desire for food, more food. There is a hidden hunger in our inner being which cannot be satisfied by physical food. My thoughts here is, how come we satisfy our physical hunger, but fail to realize our Spirit needs to be fed as well? The only way you are going to be fed spiritually is by picking up the Word of God daily and feasting at His table. My favorite time is first thing in the morning. By leaving your bible open on your counter in the kitchen it will remind you to pick up the Word and read it. Remember, we must pick up our cross daily and follow Him. I cannot tell you how thrilling it is to read His Word and every time He gives me a new revelation, it truly feeds my soul . . . An alternative for overeating is to feed yourself spiritually and that inner groaning will disappear. Okay, go ahead and feed yourself physically, I didn't mean you had to fast, but balance your physical being with your spiritual being. Fifteen to twenty minutes in the morning and perhaps another few before you shut your eyes for the night, will give you an inner peace and glow you have never experienced before. You cannot give out what you do not have inside you. Is Praise the Lord coming out of your inner being?

Feed from the Table of the Lord for inner peace and that empty cavity that can never be satisfied by food will leave!

Jesus has a table spread where the saints of God are led, He invites His Chosen People come and dine! Take the time to ask Jesus into your heart today, so you will be present at His Banqueting Table!

I hope you have enjoyed this trip with me here at my house in Lake Helen, FL and I will be awaiting the good news, that you have tried my ideas and won the Battle of the Bulge! It worked for me, it will work for you.

Here are some tips to help you along the way:

START YOUR PLAN THE NIGHT BEFORE

Decide your meals for the day.

DON'T CONSUME TO PRICE RAISING GIMMICKS, CHEAPER CEREALS ARE OFTEN NUTRITIONALLY SUPERIOR. (don't be consumed by such as, all natural,fortified with 100% of 10 essential vitamins, no preservatives, no added sugar, high fiber—missing the fact that the cereal is also high in fat, calories, natural sources of sugar and or salt.)

AVOID LONG ADDITIONS OF INGREDIENTS. The shorter the list, the better and the more nutritious the product.

SUGARS—AVOID PRODUCTS IN WHICH SUGAR OR HONEY, CORN SYRUP, FRUCTOSE OR MOLASSES IS LISTED AS THE FIRST INGREDIENT. (This could mean as much as 4 teaspoons of sugar in a one ounce bowl of cereal.)

MILK CONTAINS SODIUM—AVOID CEREALS WITH LARGE AMOUNTS OF SODIUM.

NO REASON TO BUY CEREALS WITH 100% PERCENT VITAMINS AND MINERALS.

BEWARE OF BHA and BHT PRESERVATIVES (Could indicate cancer-inhibiting properties and that BHT also inhibits the growth of viruses. If these or other preservatives are used, the label must say so.)

LIQUIDS—Very necessary.

AVOID CALORIE LADEN SWEETS. SOFT DRINKS HIGH IN SODIUM—hold water in your body and it may mask your progress in losing fat.

MIXED BLESSINGS—alcohol, caffeine in coffee, tea and other beverages is a mixed blessing. Stimulant that can raise your metabolic rate, increasing the amount of calories your body uses up. On other hand, these stimulants can lower blood sugar and speed the return of hunger sensations. 2 cups of coffee or tea, per day, no more.

SERVE YOURSELF ON A SMALL PLATE.

BUY PLAIN YOGURT

THINK HIGH FIBER

SUBSTITUTE SKIM MILK FOR WHOLE MILK

RATHER THAN SYRUP USE FRUIT OR SMEAR OF JAM TO
SWEETEN PANCAKES

BUY UNSWEETENED FRUIT JUICES AND APPLESAUCE

SERIOUSLY SPEAKING . . .

Low calorie diets are dangerous.

- . You lose water
- . Loss of protein
- . Causes you to burn Glycogen (Glycogen is stored sugar without which you would lose energy) Glycogen has each pound holding 3-4 lbs. water.
- . The only thing you accomplish is temporary weight loss.

RED FLAG UP AHEAD!

REPLACEMENT OF GLYCOGEN IS NECESSARY—EMERGENCY SUPPLY IS NEEDED TO ASSURE YOUR BRAIN OF THE SUGAR IT NEEDS TO OPERATE PROPERLY. (Perhaps this could be the cause of Alzheimer's since many seniors do not eat nutritional meals.)

Flabby arms and thighs? Low-calorie diet spurs loss of protein from your muscles. Now comes Mr. Diet Fatigue and no longer do you want to work out at the gym. Exercise is the only thing that will compensate for this loss! WORK OUT!

Losing weight fast will not be as successful. How many times have you heard people say, "I'm at a plateau, I can't seem to lose any more and so they return to their old ways and regain the weight. Exercise will cause you to lose fat, not muscle or water.

SLOW ME DOWN LORD, I'SA GOING TOO FAST, I CAN'T SEE MY BROTHER WHEN HE GOES PAST. (An old spiritual expression)

EXERCISE will cause you to maintain your desired weight and it will stay "off."

TAKE YOUR MASK OFF—SEE THE TRUTH

SLOW LOSS OF WEIGHT IS THE SECRET TO SUCCESS!

Author's Contact Information

ritaaramsey@aol.com
635 Sidney Drive
Lake Helen, FL 32744

www.ingramcontent.com/pod-product-compliance
Lightning Source LLC
Chambersburg PA
CBHW020407290526
45785CB00005B/2461